Intermittent Fasting Made Easy

A Beginner's Guide to Weight Loss and Improved Metabolic Health

Dr. David D. Reid

<u>Table of Content</u>

INTRODUCTION

- Definition and explanation of intermittent fasting
- Brief history of fasting and its health benefits
- Types of intermittent fasting

CHAPTER 1: HOW INTERMITTENT FASTING WORKS

- The science behind intermittent fasting and its effects on the body
- How it affects hormones and metabolism
- Comparison to traditional calorie-restricted diets

Chapter 2: GETTING STARTED WITH INTERMITTENT FASTING

- How to prepare for intermittent fasting
- Choosing the right type of intermittent fasting for you
- Creating a fasting schedule that works with your lifestyle

CHAPTER 3: OVERCOMING COMMON CHALLENGES

- Hunger and cravings during fasting periods
- Social situations and meal planning
- Sticking to a fasting routine

CHAPTER 4: THE BENEFITS OF INTERMITTENT FASTING

- Weight loss and improved body composition
- Improved metabolic health markers
- Increased energy and focus

CHAPTER 5: THE ROLE OF EXERCISE IN INTERMITTENT FASTING

- How to exercise during fasting periods
- Benefits of combining intermittent fasting and exercise
- Sample exercise routines for intermittent fasting

CHAPTER 6: ADVANCED TOPIC IN INTERMITTENT FASTING

- Longer fasting periods and multi-day fasts

- Intermittent fasting for athletes and active individuals
- Combining intermittent fasting with other diets or lifestyle changes

CHAPTER 7: TROUBLE SHOOTING AND FAQS

- Common questions and concerns about intermittent fasting
- Troubleshooting tips for common issues
- Final advice and resources for success with intermittent fasting

"FASTING IS THE SINGLE GREATEST NATURAL HEALING THERAPY. IT IS NATURE'S ANCIENT, UNIVERSAL 'REMEDY' FOR MANY PROBLEM."

INTRODUCTION

Intermittent Fasting (IF) is a prominent dietary technique that has garnered a lot of recognition in recent years. It is a dietary behavior that includes intermittent intervals of fasting and feasting. Unlike conventional regimens that require calorie tracking or dietary restrictions, intermittent fasting concentrates on when to consume rather than what to eat. We will examine the description and explanation of intermittent fasting, its short background, and its potential health advantages. We will also examine the different kinds of intermittent fasting.

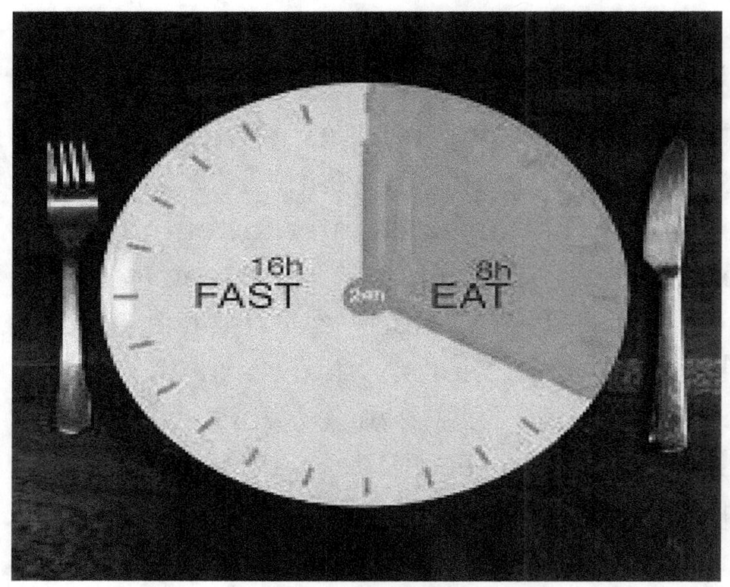

Intermittent fasting is a dietary behavior that includes alternating between intervals of fasting and consumption. During the fasting period, one restricts calorie consumption or abstains from consuming food completely, while during the feeding period, one consumes regular meals. There are several methods to practice intermittent fasting, but the most popular ones are the 16/8 approach, the 5:2 diet, and alternate-day fasting.

Fasting has been performed for millennia for different reasons, including religious, spiritual, and societal objectives. In recent years, scientific research has cast light on the potential health advantages of fasting, including weight reduction, enhanced insulin sensitivity, decreased inflammation, and increased longevity. Intermittent fasting has surfaced as a popular dietary technique due to its potential health advantages and adaptability.

Varieties of Intermittent Fasting

There are several kinds of intermittent fasting, but the most prevalent ones are the 16/8 technique, the 5:2 diet, and alternate-day fasting. The 16/8 technique includes restricting consuming to an 8-hour interval and abstaining for the remaining 16 hours. The 5:2 plan includes ingesting a regular meal for five days and restricting calorie consumption to 500-600 calories for two non-consecutive days. Alternate-day fasting includes abstaining for 24 hours every other day.

Intermittent fasting is a prevalent dietary technique that includes overlapping intervals of fasting and consumption. It has acquired recognition due to its potential health advantages and versatility. In the next portions, we will examine the different kinds of intermittent fasting in detail and their prospective advantages.

CHAPTER 1: HOW INTERMITTENT FASTING WORKS

There's a ton of tremendously encouraging intermittent fasting (IF) research done on obese rodents. They drop weight, and their blood pressure, triglycerides, and blood glucose improve but they're rodents. Research in people, almost across the board, has shown that IF is safe and successful, but really no more effective than any other regimen. In addition, many individuals find it challenging to fast.

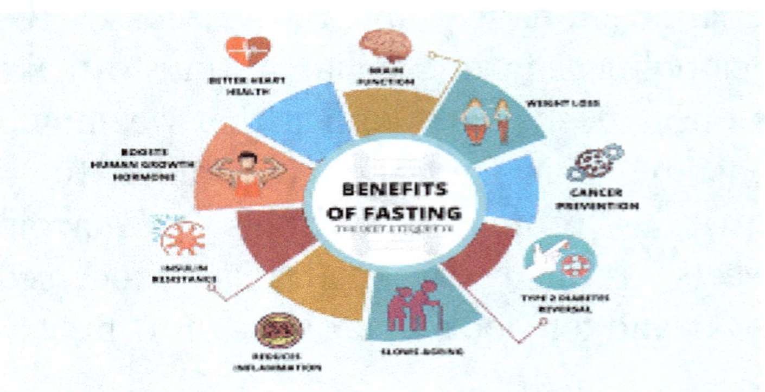

But an increasing amount of evidence indicates that the duration of the fast is important, and can make IF a more practical, sustainable, and successful strategy for weight reduction, as well as for diabetes protection.

The background on intermittent fasting

IF as a weight loss approach has been around in various forms for ages but was highly popularized in 2012.

In the Obesity Code, Fung successfully integrates plenty of research, his professional experience, and reasonable nutrition guidance, and also discusses the sociopolitical factors collaborating to make us obese. He is very explicit that we should consume more fruits and vegetables, fiber, nutritious protein, and lipids, and avoid sweets, refined carbohydrates, processed foods, and for God's sake, cease munching.

Intermittent fasting can assist weight loss. The food we consume is broken down by enzymes in our intestines and ultimately winds up as compounds in our circulation. Carbohydrates, specifically sweets and processed carbohydrates (think white flour and rice), are rapidly broken down into sugar, which our cells use for energy. If our cells don't use it all, we retain it in our fat cells as, well, fat. But sugar can only reach our cells with insulin, a hormone produced in the pancreas. Insulin transports sugar into the adipose cells and holds it there.

Between meals, as long as we don't graze, our insulin levels will go down and our fat cells can then discharge their accumulated sugar, to be used as energy. We drop weight if we let our insulin levels go down. The entire concept of IF is to enable the insulin levels to go down far enough and for long enough that we burn off our weight.

Intermittent fasting can be hard... but maybe it doesn't have to be

Original human studies that compared fasting every other day to consuming less every day revealed that both worked similarly for weight reduction, though individuals struggled with the fasting days. So, it's very reasonable to choose a decreased-calorie plant-based, Mediterranean-style diet. But research suggests that not all IF approaches are the same, and some IF diets are indeed effective and sustainable, especially when combined with a nutritious plant-based diet.

We have developed to be in harmony with the day/night pattern, i.e., a circadian schedule. Our metabolism has evolved to daylight sustenance, nocturnal slumber. Nighttime snacking is well correlated with a greater chance of obesity, as well as diabetes.

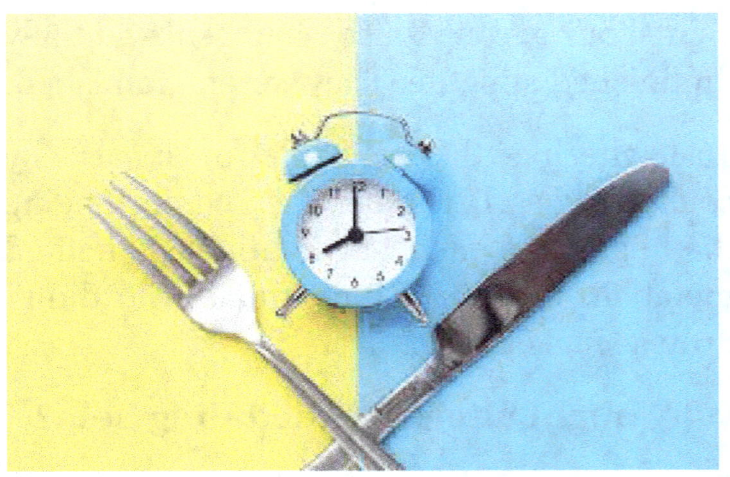

Based on this, researchers performed a survey with a small sample of heavy males with prediabetes. They compared a type of intermittent fasting termed "early time-restricted nutrition," where all meals were squeezed into an early eight-hour stretch of the day (7 am to 3 pm), or spaced out over 12 hours (between 7 am and 7 pm). Both groups maintained their weight (did not gain or lose) but after five weeks, the eight-hour group had dramatically lower insulin levels and substantially increased insulin sensitivity, as well as significantly lower blood pressure. The greatest part? The eight-hour group also had substantially diminished appetite. They weren't famished.

Just altering the schedule of meals, by consuming earlier in the day and prolonging the nighttime fast, substantially benefited metabolism even in individuals who didn't drop a single pound.

Why might altering scheduling help?

But why does merely altering the schedule of our meals to enable fasting make a difference in our bodies? An in-depth examination of the science of IF recently published in the New England Journal of Medicine provides some insight. Fasting is evolutionarily ingrained within our metabolism, activating several important biological processes. Changing the transition from a fueled to fasting condition does more than help us expend calories and drop weight.

The researchers combed through dozens of animal and human studies to explain how simple fasting improves metabolism, lowers blood sugar levels; lessens inflammation, which improves a range of health issues from arthritic pain to asthma; and even helps clear out toxins and damaged cells, which lowers risk for cancer and enhances brain function.

So, is intermittent fasting as wonderful as it sounds?

According to metabolic experts says "There is evidence to suggest that the circadian rhythm fasting approach, where meals are restricted to an eight to 10-hour period of the daytime, is effective." But still, encourages people "use a dietary strategy that works for them and is sustainable to them."

So, here's the situation. There is some solid scientific evidence indicating that circadian rhythm fasting, when combined with a healthy diet and lifestyle, can be a particularly successful strategy for weight reduction, especially for individuals at risk for diabetes. (However, people with established diabetes or who are on medications for diabetes, people with a history of eating disorders like anorexia and bulimia, and expectant or breastfeeding women should not attempt intermittent fasting unless under the careful supervision of a physician who can observe them.)

Avoid sweets and processed carbohydrates. Instead, consume fruits, vegetables, legumes, lentils, whole cereals, lean proteins, and healthy lipids (a reasonable, plant-based, Mediterranean-style diet) (a sensible, plant-based, Mediterranean-style diet).

Let your body eliminate fat between meals. Don't graze. Be moving throughout your day. Improve muscular tone.

Contemplate a straightforward type of intermittent fasting. Restrict the hours of the day when you consume, and for optimal impact, make it earlier in the day (between 7 am to 3 pm, or even 10 am to 6 pm, but absolutely not in the evening before bed)

Prevent nibbling or consuming at nightfall, all the time.

Intermittent fasting (IF) has been getting recognition as a nutritional approach for weight reduction and enhancing metabolic health. The procedure includes restraining food consumption for a defined duration, which results in alternating periods of fasting and feasting. Several studies have investigated the potential impacts of intermittent fasting on hormones and metabolism, and the findings have been encouraging.

Insulin

Insulin is a hormone generated by the pancreas that modulates blood sugar levels in the body. Insulin resistance, which is distinguished by the body's incapacity to respond to insulin, is a primary cause of type 2 diabetes. Intermittent fasting has been shown to increase insulin sensitivity, which can help stabilize blood sugar levels and decrease the chance of developing diabetes.

During the fasting interval, insulin levels in the body diminish, and the body depends on conserved glycogen for energy. This results in reduced blood sugar levels and encourages the decomposition of stored fat for energy. When the grazing period restarts, the body utilizes the ingested food to replenish its energy reserves and generates insulin to regulate blood sugar levels.

Development hormone

Growth hormone (GH) is generated by the pituitary gland and is necessary for growth and development, muscular construction, and fat reduction. GH production is controlled by the body's circadian schedule, with the greatest amounts generated during slumber. Intermittent fasting has been shown to increase GH production, resulting in enhanced body composition and metabolism.

One research investigated the impacts of alternate-day fasting on GH production in normal-weight individuals. The findings revealed that GH levels increased substantially during the fasting period and remained elevated for up to 24 hours after the feeding period restarted. This indicates that intermittent fasting can increase GH generation and enhance metabolic health.

Cortisol

Cortisol is a stress hormone that is generated by the adrenal glands in reaction to stress. Elevated cortisol levels are correlated with heightened inflammation, weight growth, and a greater chance of contracting chronic illnesses. Intermittent fasting has been shown to decrease cortisol levels, resulting in enhanced cardiovascular health.

One research investigated the impacts of alternate-day fasting on cortisol levels in healthy individuals. The findings revealed that cortisol levels decreased substantially during the fasting interval, indicating that intermittent fasting can reduce stress and enhance cardiovascular health.

Norepinephrine

Norepinephrine is a hormone generated by the adrenal glands and functions as a neurotransmitter in the central nervous system. It is responsible for increasing energy levels, enhancing concentration, and encouraging fat metabolism. Intermittent fasting has been shown to increase norepinephrine levels, resulting in enhanced cardiovascular health.

An expert investigated the impacts of alternate-day fasting on norepinephrine levels in normal-weight individuals. The findings revealed that norepinephrine levels increased substantially during the fasting interval, indicating that intermittent fasting can encourage fat metabolism and enhance metabolic health.

Leptin

Leptin is a hormone generated by adipose cells that modulates appetite and metabolism. Elevated amounts of leptin are associated with diminished appetite and increased metabolism, while low levels are associated with increased hunger and decreased metabolism. Intermittent fasting may decrease leptin levels, resulting in enhanced cardiovascular health.

Leptin levels decreased substantially during the fasting period, indicating that intermittent fasting can increase the body's sensitivity to hunger impulses and encourage weight reduction.

Mitochondrial rate

Metabolic rate is the pace at which the body consumes nutrients for energy. Intermittent fasting can increase metabolic rate, resulting in increased weight reduction and cardiovascular health. Metabolic rate increased substantially during the fasting interval, resulting in enhanced weight reduction and metabolic health.

Chapter 2: GETTING STARTED WITH INTERMITTENT FASTING

Intermittent fasting is a scheduled strategy for consuming. Before beginning, a person can prepare by figuring out why they want to fast, what type of fast they plan to follow, what type of food plan suits them best, and so on.

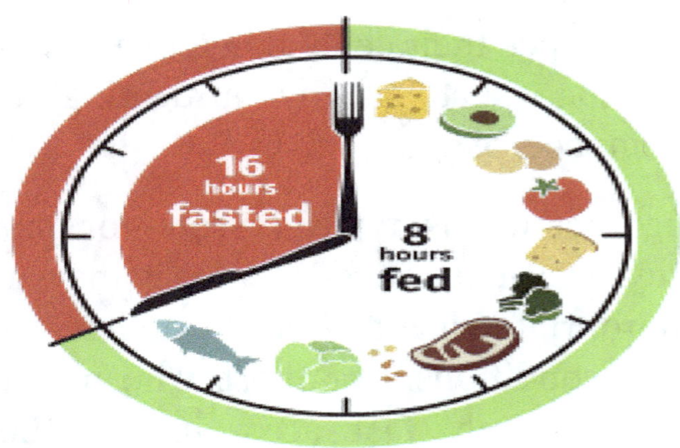

Intermittent fasting includes alternating between periods of consuming and periods of abstaining. It does not stipulate which meals to ingest or avoid but recommends a timeframe in which to consume sustenance.

At first, individuals may find it challenging to consume during a brief interval of time each day or to alternate between days of eating and not eating.

Intermittent fasting is a prevalent technique that individuals use to:

- Streamline their existence
- Reduce weight
- Enhance their general health and well-being, such as by mitigating the impacts of aging

Though fasting is typically safe for most healthy, well-nourished people, it may not be appropriate for individuals who have any medical conditions. For those who may be able to securely fast according to their doctor, the following suggestions hope to help make the experience as simple and beneficial as feasible.

Identify specific objectives

Generally, an individual who begins intermittent fasting has a purpose in mind. It may be to reduce weight, improve general health, or enhance digestive health. A person's eventual objective will help them determine the most appropriate fasting technique and figure out how many calories and nutrition they need to consume.

Select the technique

An individual may attempt numerous prospective techniques when fasting for health purposes. They should select a strategy that matches their inclinations and that they believe they can adhere to.

A few of the more prevalent fasting regimens are:

- Intermittent fasting or time-restricted feeding
- Alternate-day fasting

Generally, a person should persist with one fasting technique for a month or longer to see whether it works for them before attempting a different method. Anyone who has a medical condition should contact a healthcare practitioner before commencing any fasting technique. Fasting is not a secure choice for some individuals.

When choosing a technique, a person should consider that they do not need to consume a certain quantity or variety of food or forgo certain items completely. An individual can consume what they want when following an intermittent fasting strategy.

However, to achieve health and weight management objectives, it is a good plan to follow a balanced, high protein, high fiber, vegetable-rich diet during dining intervals.

Eating only meals that lack advantageous nutrition during dining intervals can impede healthy development. It is also extremely essential to consume loads of water or other no-calorie refreshments throughout fasting intervals.

Periodic starvation

This framework includes fasting within specified time intervals, such as twice per week, as with the Consume Stop Eat strategy and the 5:2 technique.

Consume Cease Eat

Brad Pilon developed Eat Stop Eat, a fasting technique that includes consuming nothing for 24 hours twice a week. It does not matter on which days a person fasts or even when they commence. The only restriction is that fasting must last for 24 hours and occur on nonconsecutive days.

Individuals who do not consume for 24 hours will likely become very famished. Consuming Cease Food may not be the ideal technique for individuals who are inexperienced with fasting. An individual should contact a doctor or registered nutritionist before beginning a fasting strategy like this one.

5:2 technique

An individual on the 5:2 approach consumes 500–600 calories 2 days each week, on either consecutive or non-consecutive days, depending on the particular schedule.

Time-restricted feeding

Programs such as the Warrior Diet and the 16/8 or 14/10 approach are considered time-restricted eating, in which a person consumes nutrients only within specified intervals of time throughout the day.

Spartan Diet

Ori Hofmekler is the inventor of the Warrior Plan, which involves consuming very little for 20 hours each day. An individual refraining in this manner consumes all their average food consumption in the remaining 4 hours.

Consuming a whole day's worth of food in such a brief period can make a person's stomach quite uncomfortable. This is a more intense starvation technique. As with Eat Stop Eat, a person new to fasting may not want to commence with this technique and should contact a doctor before attempting it.

Leangains

Martin Berkhan developed Leangains for weightlifters, but it has become popular among other people who are interested in dieting as well. Unlike Consume Stop Eat and the Warrior Program, fasting for Leangains includes much shorter intervals.

For example, males who choose the Leangains technique fast for 16 hours and then consume what they want for the remaining 8 hours of the day. Females fast for 14 hours and consume what they want for the remaining 10 hours of the day.

During the fast, a person must avoid consuming any food but can consume as many no-calorie beverages as they like.

16:8 Technique of intermittent fasting

16:8 Intermittent fasting provides for a fast spanning 16 hours per day, with all meals consumed during the remaining 8 hours. The following periods for consuming are prevalent with this fasting strategy, with overnight hours included in the fasting time:

- 9 a.m. to 5 p.m.
- 10 a.m. to 6 p.m. or noon to 8 p.m.
- Alternate-day fasting

Some individuals fast on alternate days to help improve blood sugar or cholesterol levels or to help control their weight.

Some alternate-day fasting routines incorporate a third day of fasting each week. For the remainder of the week, a person consumes only the amount of calories they expend during the day. Over time, this produces a calorie imbalance that enables the individual to drop weight if that is their objective.

Calculate calorie requirements

There are no intrinsic nutritional restrictions when intermittent fasting, but this does not mean that calories do not matter.

Individuals who are working with a doctor or nutritionist to control their weight need to establish a calorie imbalance, which means ingesting fewer calories than they use. Individuals who are seeking to acquire weight need to consume more calories than they use.

Many resources are available to help a person figure out their calorie requirements and determine how many calories they should consume each day to acquire, reduce, or maintain weight.

A person could also contact a healthcare practitioner or nutritionist for assistance on how many calories they need. A professional can help a person determine the best meals for them and discover an overall healthful method to reduce weight.

Figure out a food schedule

A person interested in dropping or gaining weight may find it beneficial to prepare what they are going to consume during the day or week.

Food preparation does not need to be excessively restrictive. It considers calorie consumption and incorporates appropriate nutrition into the diet. For example, the Centers for Disease Control and Prevention (CDC) recommends the MyPlatePlan, which concentrates on displaying a person's dietary category objectives for each day.

Food preparation offers many advantages, such as helping a person adhere to their calorie tally and ensuring they have the necessary ingredients on hand for recipes, simple dinners, and munchies. As a potential benefit, dinner preparation could save money if it helps people discard less food.

Make the calories matter

Not all nutrients are the same. Although these fasting techniques do not restrict the number of calories a person consumes during feeding periods, it is important to consider the nutritional worth of the food.

In general, a person should strive to consume nutrient-dense meals or foods with a large number of nutrients per calorie. They may not have to forsake less nutritious food completely, but they should still exercise temperance and concentrate on more nutritional choices to receive the most benefits.

How efficient is intermittent fasting?

Fasting has several impacts on a person's body:

- ✓ Fasting reduces amounts of insulin, making it simpler for the body to use stored fat.
- ✓ It lowers blood sugar, blood pressure, and inflammatory levels.

- ✓ It may affect the expression of certain genes, which can help the body safeguard itself from illness and encourage longevity.
- ✓ It increases human growth hormone levels, which can help the body use body waste and build muscle.

According to a 2018 analysis of studies , calorie restriction, and intermittent fasting can help the body initiate a mending process called autophagy, which essentially means that the body digests or recycles old or injured cell components.

Fasting extends back to prehistoric humans, who often went hours or days between meals because acquiring sustenance was challenging. The human body acclimated to this manner of eating, enabling prolonged intervals to elapse between-meal consumption times.

Intermittent fasting can be very beneficial for weight management. The practice may serve as a beneficial instrument in the management of obesity, though more long-term studies are required.

Evidence also indicates that fasting has a variety of other advantages.

It may be beneficial for controlling metabolic syndrome and diabetes. It may help preserve neural activity. Fasting may be advantageous in managing intestinal health conditions such as irritable bowel syndrome, although more research is required. It may even lengthen the life span.

Side consequences

For a healthy individual, intermittent fasting has few potential adverse effects.

When a person first begins fasting, they may feel slightly physically and psychologically lethargic as their body changes. After the transition, most individuals go back to functioning as they did before.

However, individuals with medical conditions should contact their doctor before commencing any fasting regimen. Individuals who are particularly at risk of deleterious consequences from fasting and who may require additional medical supervision include those who:

- ✓ Are breastfeeding
- ✓ Are pregnant

Benefits on activity

For healthy individuals, intermittent fasting should not impact their ability to exercise, except during the period when their body is transitioning to the new dietary timetable. After the acclimation period, a person should not experience any detrimental impacts on their exercise regimen as a consequence of fasting.

Those concerned about losing muscle while fasting should be sure to consume enough protein during feeding periods and participate in resistance exercises frequently. By keeping protein consumption up, a person is less likely to lose muscular density from starvation.

Researchers investigated the impact on males who participated in both resistance exercise and intermittent fasting. They discovered that the participants dropped general body weight and maintained their muscular mass by following the 16:8 fasting strategy.

However, more research is essential to completely comprehend all the impacts of intermittent fasting on the body.

Fasting is a necessary component of the human life cycle. Most people have fasted unwittingly throughout their lifetimes by having an early supper and foregoing breakfast the next day. More regimented techniques may work well for some individuals.

It is essential to bear in mind that although a person does not need to exclude certain items from their diet while fasting, they should strive to consume a balanced diet high in protein, fiber, fruits, and vegetables. It is also essential to consume plenty of reduced-calorie or no-calorie beverages.

Though the typical person will likely experience few or no adverse effects from fasting, people who have certain medical conditions or take certain medications should contact their doctor before attempting a fasting strategy.

There are so many different methods to do IF, and that's a wonderful thing. If this is something you're interested in doing, you can discover the strategy that will work best with your lifestyle, which increases the possibilities of success.

CHAPTER 3: OVERCOMING COMMON CHALLENGES

With the trend of diets, more individuals are practicing intermittent fasting to reduce weight. It may be working out great for them, but there is also a portion of individuals who feel trapped in scheduled meals and eating periods, particularly when they feel like eating anything. Have you ever found yourself yearning while intermittent fasting? Well, sure, hunger is a feature of intermittent fasting, but it can be managed.

If you have been pondering partaking in intermittent fasting, nevertheless, you are unable to effectively do so since you tend to succumb to food cravings. But there are a few established strategies which will assist you fast without any desired disruptions."

Increase your water intake

Along with keeping you hydrated, water assists in regularizing your appetite cycle. There are instances when you may sense that you are hungry, yet, your body may merely be low on water. People, who prefer to drink more water during the day, have claimed to feel less hungry. Water also assists in improved absorption of your diet.

Consume protein-rich meals

Protein-rich meals aid in stabilizing blood sugar levels and reducing appetite hormones which makes you feel less hungry and helps you manage cravings. Protein also helps you retain lean muscle which is vital for weight reduction.

Increase fiber intake

Fiber is widely recognized to aid in digestion. Fiber-rich meals control blood sugar levels in the body and also supply sustenance to healthy bacteria in the stomach which aid in effectively absorbing nutrients from the ingested food, making you feel less hungry.

Eat slowly

When you eat too rapidly, it takes your mind some time to recognize that your stomach is full, and as a consequence of which, most individuals tend to eat more than needed and give into cravings. Instead, eat slowly and focus on every mouthful which will help you restrict your food consumption.

Keep yourself occupied

In a lot of instances, you may believe that you are hungry; however, the fact is that you are merely bored and are feeling desires. While practicing intermittent fasting, it is vital that you keep yourself active and diverted from food.

Other ideas to keep in mind to control cravings: 1. Follow a balanced diet plan to ensure that you acquire all the nutrients since sometimes yearning is the consequence of a lack of nourishment in the body.

2. Along with eating healthily, eat at regular intervals. Your blood sugar levels may decrease if you miss a meal, which can induce cravings.

3. There's no requirement to avoid calories totally while practicing intermittent fasting. But make sure when you eat, you add healthy alternatives of calories and consume in moderation.

4. Chewing gum is a terrific strategy to lower your appetite, which might keep you from overeating and can put a complete stop to your desires.

5. Understand the difference between fasting and starvation. Therefore, if your desires are prompted by hunger, make sure you eat something. Otherwise, it might have the opposite effect.

Social activities and food preparation may be an issue for people who follow an IF schedule. However, with good preparation and communication, it is easy to keep an IF schedule while enjoying social activities and meals with friends and family.

Communicate your IF plan

It might be beneficial to express your IF strategy to your friends or family members in advance of social activities. Let them know that you are fasting during specified hours, and ask if they can accommodate your eating plan. Most people will be supportive and understanding, and some may even join you in fasting.

Adjust your fasting schedule

If you know you will be attending a social gathering or going out for a meal, prepare ahead by altering your fasting schedule. For example, if you generally fast from 8 pm to 12 pm the following day, you may alter your schedule to fast from 4 pm to 12 pm the next day. This would enable you to share a dinner with friends or family without disturbing your IF regimen.

Choose the correct foods

When arranging meals for social occasions, consider items that are in keeping with your

IF objectives. Select meals that are abundant in protein, healthy fats, and fiber, which can help keep you satisfied for longer times. Foods that are low in calories, like vegetables, are also terrific selections.

Be aware of portion sizes

It might be tempting to indulge in huge servings on social occasions, but it's crucial to be cautious of portion proportions. Remember that the purpose of IF is to lower total calorie consumption, so try to avoid overeating. If you do indulge, think prolonging your fasting time the following day to compensate for the increased calories.

Stay hydrated

Drinking water is vital during IF to keep your body hydrated and fend off hunger sensations. Before attending social gatherings, drink enough water to make you feel full and pleased. You might also carry a water bottle with you to events to ensure you keep hydrated throughout the day.

Avoid alcohol

Alcohol might disturb your fasting schedule and impede weight reduction objectives. If you prefer to drink, choose low-calorie beverages such as vodka and soda or light beer. Remember to drink in moderation and remain hydrated by alternating alcoholic drinks with water.

Be flexible

Intermittent fasting should not be considered a rigorous diet that cannot be changed to meet social occasions. Being flexible with your fasting schedule and eating habits may help you maintain a healthy connection with food while still enjoying social occasions. Don't be too harsh on yourself if you break your IF regimen sometimes. Instead, concentrate on getting back on track as quickly as possible.

Social activities and meal preparation may be a struggle while following an IF schedule, but with appropriate planning and communication, it is possible to keep your routine while still enjoying social gatherings and dinners with friends and family. Remember to explain your IF strategy, change your fasting schedule as required, pick the correct meals, be cautious of portion sizes, remain hydrated, avoid alcohol, and be flexible. With these strategies, you may enjoy social activities while still accomplishing your IF objectives.

Sticking to a fasting practice may be tough, particularly for those new to intermittent fasting (IF). However, with the correct mentality, methods, and support, it is feasible to build a sustained and productive fasting regimen.

Here are some ideas for adhering to a fasting routine:

Set a reasonable objective

Setting a reasonable goal is the first step in building a sustained fasting regimen. It's crucial to establish a fasting plan that is feasible and fits into your lifestyle. For example, if you are new to IF, you may want to start with a 12-hour fast and progressively expand the fasting window to 14 or 16 hours as you get more comfortable.

Plan ahead

Planning ahead is crucial to adhere to a fasting practice. Before commencing your fast, make sure you have nutritious and substantial meals and snacks accessible to break your fast. This can assist you to avoid making poor meal choices due to hunger or lack of preparation. You may also structure your fasting schedule around social engagements or work responsibilities to make it simpler to adhere to.

Keep busy

Keeping oneself active during a fast will help distract you from hunger sensations and keep you on track. Engage in things that keep you intellectually and physically active, such as going for a walk, performing yoga, or reading a book.

Find a support system

Having a support system might be useful in adhering to a fasting habit. Consider joining an online fasting group or finding a fasting companion who can give inspiration and support. You may also seek help from a certified dietician or a healthcare practitioner.

Listen to your body

It's vital to listen to your body and alter your fasting schedule appropriately. If you feel weak or dizzy during a fast, try breaking it early or decreasing the fasting window. It's also vital to pay attention to how your body reacts to various kinds of food and change your diet appropriately.

Practice self-compassion

Intermittent fasting is not a one-size-fits-all technique, and it's natural to suffer setbacks or obstacles along the road. Practice self-compassion and don't be too harsh on yourself if you break your fast or depart from your schedule. Instead, concentrate on getting back on track and continue working towards your objectives.

Adhering to a fasting habit involves dedication, strategy, and support. By establishing a realistic goal, preparing ahead, staying hydrated, keeping active, finding a support system, listening to your body, and practicing self-compassion, you may develop a sustainable and successful fasting pattern that works for you. Remember, consistency is crucial, and with time and experience, fasting may become a natural and joyful part of your daily.

CHAPTER 4: THE BENEFITS OF INTERMITTENT FASTING

Why would someone select this manner of eating against a regular diet, such as adopting low carb or low fat? Some folks claim fasting offers tons of health advantages. The research so far proves the benefits of IF to the extent that it is worthwhile as a method to lose weight, manage your blood sugar, and slow down the aging process.

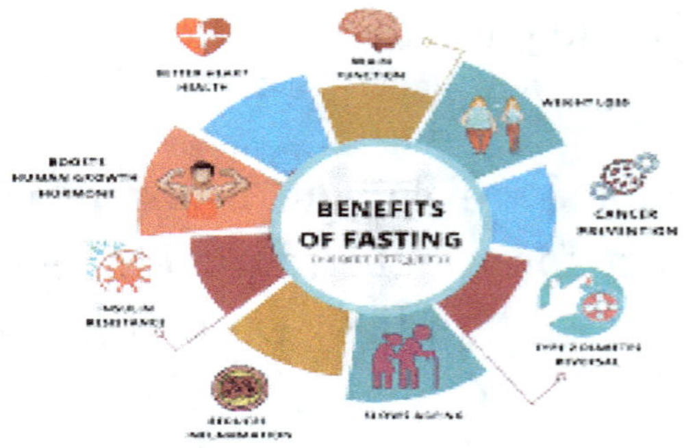

But not everyone's on board. From my standpoint and the standpoint of a lot of other people, it does tend to fall into the next fad diet category. A lot of the evidence is disputed, and many experiments were done on animals have not yet been duplicated in humans. For every study that shows there's no change, there are some studies that show maybe there is an improvement.

Weight Loss

Most individuals start IF to reduce weight. And that assertion appears to hold up, at least in the near run. IF may help with weight reduction for overweight or obese persons. IF helps patients shed up to 13 percent of their weight.

That's obviously excellent news if you're trying to fast for weight reduction, but the fact that those studies were short-term means it's uncertain whether IF is sustainable and can help you keep off excess pounds in the long run.

What's more, not all studies have indicated IF resulted in weight reduction. Research published in September 2020 with 116 overweight or obese persons who ate between the hours of 12 and 8 p.m. for 12 weeks revealed that they did not have substantially higher weight reduction than the control group.

The second catch: The amount of weight loss doesn't appear to be much higher than what you'd anticipate from another calorie-restricted diet. Equivalent quantities of weight and fat reduction were achieved by IF and continuous energy restriction, such as a low-calorie diet. And depending on how many calories you're consuming each day, you may even wind up gaining weight. After all, the diet doesn't limit high-calorie meals or overall calories – it merely restricts when you may eat.

When the diet is done correctly, IF may be as successful as conventional calorie restriction, Lowden adds. Some individuals, particularly busy people who don't have time to commit to meal preparation, could even find a time-restricted diet simpler to follow than something like the keto diet or the paleo diet.

Reduced Blood Pressure

IF may help decrease high blood pressure in the near term. 16:8 substantially lowered systolic blood pressure in the 23 study participants. Systolic blood pressure is the highest number in your blood pressure measurement and shows the power of the heart on your artery walls each time it beats.

The association between lower systolic blood pressure and IF exists in both animal and human research. IF led to significantly bigger decreases in systolic blood pressure than another diet that didn't contain set meal periods.

Having healthy blood pressure is vital, excessive levels may affect your heart, brain, kidneys, and eyes.

But so far the evidence reveals that these blood pressure advantages persist just when someone is trying IF. Once the diet ended and participants resumed eating as was typical for them, researchers discovered that blood pressure readings reverted to their original levels.

Reduced Inflammation

Animal research shows that both IF and general calorie restriction may lower inflammatory levels, while clinical trials are few and far between. My team, last year investigated a group of 50 volunteers who were fasting for Ramadan, the Muslim holiday, which requires fasting from dawn to sunset and eating overnight. We found that during the fasting phase, pro-inflammatory indicators were lower than normal, as were blood pressure, body weight, and body fat.

Lower Cholesterol

Several kinds of IF, including alternate-day fasting and 5:2, may help decrease LDL ("bad") cholesterol, among other measures of cardiometabolic health, such as blood pressure.

LDL cholesterol may enhance your risk of heart disease or stroke, according to the CDC. The researchers also discovered that IF lowered the level of triglycerides, which are lipids present in the blood that might contribute to stroke, heart attack, or heart disease.

Yet not all researchers think that IF dramatically decreases cholesterol levels

Better Outcomes for Stroke Survivors

Healthier cholesterol levels and lower blood pressure (two advantages discussed above) play a big role in helping lessen your risk of stroke. But that's not the only probable stroke-related benefit of IF. Fasting may offer a protective mechanism for the brain and increase recovery from a stroke, mainly due to IF's anti-inflammatory impact. That was the finding based on animal studies -

the researchers highlighted that human data about the effects of IF on stroke are missing.

Boosted Brain Function

IF may increase mental sharpness and attention. And there's some early evidence to support that idea: A research published in November 2021 in Molecular Psychiatry indicated that fasting every other day may increase memory. This research was done exclusively on animals, however. Intermittent fasting doesn't appear to contribute to short-term cognitive improvements among healthy individuals, but it may protect against the development of a neurological illness.

CHAPTER 5: THE ROLE OF EXERCISE IN INTERMITTENT FASTING

Many individuals are also interested in including exercise in their intermittent fasting habit, but they are not sure how to do it efficiently. We will cover the importance of exercise in intermittent fasting, how to exercise during fasting times, the advantages of combining intermittent fasting with exercise, and examples of exercise routines for intermittent fasting.

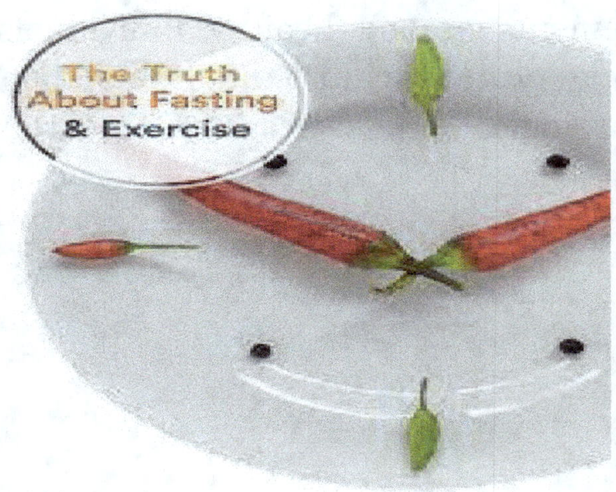

If you're attempting IF or you're fasting for other reasons and you still want to get your workouts in, there are some benefits and downsides to consider before you decide to work out in a fasted condition.

Some study reveals that exercising while fasting impacts muscle biochemistry and metabolism that's connected to insulin sensitivity and the stable maintenance of blood sugar levels.

Research also suggests eating and immediately exercising before digestion or absorption happens. This is especially critical for anybody with type 2 diabetes or metabolic syndrome.

A very interesting stuff when fasting is that your stored carbs known as glycogen are most likely exhausted, so you'll be burning more fat to power your exercise.

Does the chance to burn more fat seem like a win? Before you hop on the quickest cardio fad, there's a disadvantage.

While exercising in a fasting condition, it's conceivable that your body may start breaking down muscle to utilize protein for fuel. Plus, you're more susceptible to hitting the wall, which means you'll have less energy and not be able to work out as hard or perform as well.

Intermittent fasting and exercising long term isn't desirable. Your body depletes itself of calories and energy, which could ultimately end up slowing your metabolism.

You're fasting, should you work out?

You may burn more fat.

If fasting long term, you might slow down your metabolism.

You may not perform as effectively during exercises.

You may lose muscle mass or only be able to maintain, not gain muscle.

Getting in an efficient gym session while fasting

If you're prepared to attempt IF while maintaining your exercise regimen, there are certain things you can do to make your workout beneficial.

Think through timing

There are three factors for making your workout more successful when fasting: whether you should exercise before, during, or after the feeding window.

One typical way of IF is the 16:8 protocol. The notion relates to ingesting all meals during an 8-hour fueling window and then fasting for 16 hours.

Working out before the window is ideal for someone who performs well during exercise on an empty stomach, while during the window is better suited for someone who doesn't like to exercise on an empty stomach and also wants to capitalize on post-workout nutrition

After the window is for people who like to exercise after fueling but don't have the opportunity to do it during the eating window.

Eat the correct foods after your exercise to grow or retain muscle

The greatest option for mixing IF with exercise is to plan your exercises around your feeding times so your nutrient levels are peaked.

And if you do the heavy lifting, it's important for your body to have protein after the workout to aid with regeneration.

I suggests following up any strength exercise with carbs and roughly 20 grams of protein within 30 minutes after your session.

How can you safely exercise while fasting?

The effectiveness of any weight reduction or fitness program hinges on how safe it is to continue over time. If your ultimate aim is to lower body fat and maintain your fitness level while doing IF, you need to remain in the safe zone. Here are some professional recommendations to help you achieve exactly that.

Eat a meal close to your moderate- to high-intensity exercise

This is when mealtime comes into play. Planning a meal close to moderate- or high-intensity activity is crucial. This way your body has some glycogen resources to dip into to power your exercise.

Keep your electrolytes up

A fantastic low-calorie hydration option, is coconut water. It replenishes electrolytes, is low in calories, and tastes pretty good Gatorade and sports drinks are heavy in sugar, so avoid drinking too much of them.

Keep the intensity and duration reasonably modest

If you push yourself too hard and begin to feel dizzy or light-headed, take a rest. Listening to your body is key.

While exercising with intermittent fasting may work for some individuals, others may not feel comfortable performing any type of activity while fasting.

Check with your doctor or healthcare professional before beginning any diet or exercise regimen.

Exercising during fasting times may be tough since your body is in a condition of low energy and requires nutrition to perform efficiently. However, there are several tactics you may employ to make exercise more pleasant and pleasurable during fasting times.

It is crucial to pick the correct time to exercise. Most individuals find it simpler to exercise in the morning before breaking their fast since they have not eaten anything for many hours and their glycogen levels are depleted. This may help your body burn fat more effectively and enhance your energy levels.

It is vital to keep hydrated throughout your fast and workout program. Drink lots of water throughout the day, and try adding electrolytes to your drink to assist maintain your hydration levels.

It is vital to start carefully and gradually increase the intensity and length of your exercises. If you are new to fasting and exercise, start with low-intensity workouts such as strolling, yoga, or stretching. As your body adjusts to fasting and exercise, you may progressively increase the intensity and length of your exercises.

Combining intermittent fasting and exercise may give various advantages to your health and wellness. Here are some of the benefits of including exercise in your intermittent fasting routine:

Improved weight loss: Combining intermittent fasting and exercise will help you lose weight more successfully. Exercise may help your body burn fat more effectively while fasting can assist lower your calorie intake and encourage fat reduction.

Enhanced cellular health: Intermittent fasting and exercise may both promote cellular repair and lower oxidative stress, which can enhance your general health and reduce your risk of chronic illnesses.

Sample Exercise Routines for Intermittent Fasting

Morning stroll: Take a quick stroll in the morning before breaking your fast. Walking is a low-intensity workout that may help you burn fat and enhance your energy levels.

Yoga: Practice yoga throughout your fasting time to enhance flexibility, decrease tension, and promote relaxation.

Strength Training: Do strength training activities such as bodyweight workouts, weightlifting, or resistance bands throughout your eating intervals to develop muscle and improve overall fitness.

High-Intensity Interval Training (HIIT): Incorporate HIIT exercises into your eating intervals to burn fat and raise your metabolic rate.

Swimming: Go for a swim throughout your eating times

CHAPTER 6: ADVANCED TOPIC IN INTERMITTENT FASTING

Intermittent fasting (IF) has been a popular dietary fad in recent years because of its possible health advantages, including weight reduction, increased insulin sensitivity, and lower inflammation. However, as individuals grow more comfortable with IF, they may wish to investigate advanced themes and practices to maximize their fasting experience.

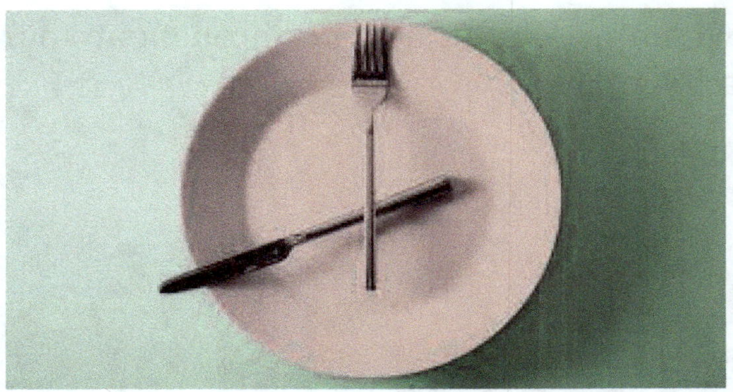

Longer fasting durations and multi-day fasts

While most people practice intermittent fasting for 16-24 hours at a time, certain individuals may choose extended fasting periods or even multi-day fasts. Extended fasting, also known as extended fasting, may vary from 24 to 72 hours or more. Multi-day fasts may continue up to several weeks, however, it is crucial to emphasize that they should only be done under the guidance of a healthcare practitioner.

Extended fasting and multi-day fasts may be tough, both physically and psychologically, but they may bring extra health advantages such as enhanced autophagy (a cellular cleansing process) and ketosis (a metabolic state where the body burns fat for fuel).

Intermittent fasting for athletes and active folks

Intermittent fasting may be tough for athletes and active persons who need to ingest enough calories and nutrients to maintain their physical activity and recuperation. However, IF may still be utilized as a strategy for weight control and general wellness.

One method is to plan the fasting phase around exercises and refill with nutrient-dense meals during the eating window. Another alternative is to integrate "fasted" exercises, which entail exercising in a fasted condition to improve fat burning and enhance insulin sensitivity.

It is vital to highlight that athletes and active persons should evaluate their energy levels and performance while fasting and alter their fasting and eating regimens appropriately.

Combining intermittent fasting with other diets or lifestyle changes

Some people may combine intermittent fasting with other diets or lifestyle modifications to further boost their health and wellness objectives. For example, some individuals may adopt a low-carbohydrate, high-fat ketogenic diet during the eating window to induce ketosis and fat burning.

Others may follow time-restricted feeding (TRF), which entails eating all meals inside a specified time frame, such as 10 am to 6 pm, to coincide with the body's circadian cycles and optimize metabolic health.

It is crucial to highlight that combining IF with other diets or lifestyle modifications should be done under the advice of a healthcare practitioner to guarantee proper nutritional intake and minimize any negative effects.

Intermittent fasting is a flexible and customized method to improve health and fitness. Advanced subjects such as prolonged fasting periods, intermittent fasting for athletes, and combining IF with other diets or lifestyle modifications may give extra rewards and difficulties for individuals looking to enhance their fasting experience. As always, it is crucial to talk with a healthcare expert before making any changes to your diet or lifestyle.

CHAPTER 7: TROUBLE SHOOTING AND FAQS

Intermittent fasting can come with its own set of challenges. Here are some common questions and concerns about intermittent fasting, as well as troubleshooting tips and final advice for success.

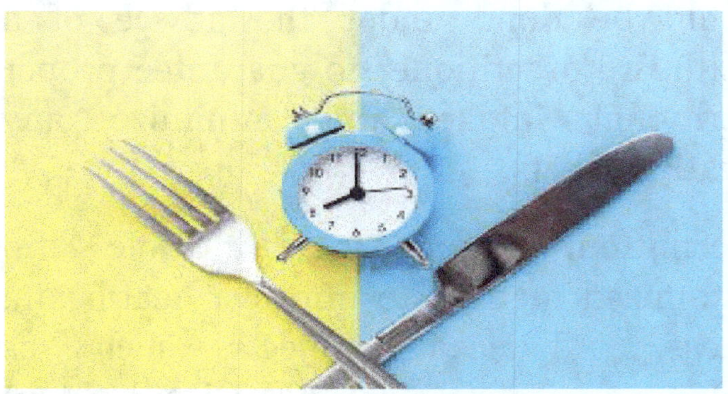

Common questions and concerns about intermittent fasting

a. Will intermittent fasting cause muscle loss?

Intermittent fasting, when done properly, should not cause muscle loss. Some studies have shown that intermittent fasting can help preserve muscle mass while promoting fat loss. It's important to ensure that you're consuming enough protein during the feeding window to support muscle growth and repair.

b. Can I still consume calories during the fasting period?

The goal of intermittent fasting is to restrict calorie intake during the fasting window to allow the body to enter a state of autophagy and promote fat burning. Consuming any calories during the fasting window, such as through snacks or beverages, can disrupt this process.

c. Can intermittent fasting be harmful to my health?

Intermittent fasting is generally safe for healthy individuals, but it's important to approach it with a sustainable and realistic mindset. Individuals with underlying health conditions, pregnant or breastfeeding women, and individuals with a history of eating disorders should seek guidance from a healthcare professional before starting intermittent fasting.

Troubleshooting tips for common issues

a. I'm feeling fatigued during the fasting period.

Fatigue during the fasting period can be caused by dehydration or nutrient deficiencies. Drinking plenty of water and consuming nutrient-dense foods during the feeding window can help alleviate fatigue.

b. I'm experiencing digestive issues during the fasting period.

Digestive issues during the fasting period may be caused by overeating during the feeding window or consuming foods that are difficult to digest. Eating smaller, more frequent meals during the feeding window and avoiding foods that trigger digestive issues can help alleviate these symptoms.

c. I'm experiencing mood swings or irritability during the fasting period.

Mood swings and irritability during the fasting period can be caused by fluctuations in blood sugar levels. Consuming nutrient-dense foods during the feeding window and avoiding high-sugar, high-carbohydrate foods can help stabilize blood sugar levels and alleviate these symptoms.

Final advice and resources for success with intermittent fasting

Intermittent fasting can be a beneficial lifestyle change for improving overall health and wellness, but it's important to approach it with a realistic and sustainable mindset. Here are some final tips and resources for success:

a. Start slowly and gradually increase fasting periods to allow the body to adjust.

b. Incorporate nutrient-dense foods and regular physical activity during the feeding window.

c. Seek guidance from a healthcare professional before starting intermittent fasting, especially if you have underlying health conditions.

d. Join online communities or seek support from a registered dietitian to stay motivated and informed.

In conclusion, intermittent fasting can be a challenging but rewarding lifestyle change. By addressing common questions and concerns, troubleshooting issues, and seeking support and resources, individuals can successfully incorporate intermittent fasting into their daily routines for improved health and wellness.